Vegetarian

Table of Contents

Book 3

Chapter 1: Sweets And Snack Options 2
Chapter 2: Week One 7
Chapter 3: Week Two 10
Chapter 4: Week Three 13
Chapter 5: Week Four 16
Chapter 6: Week Five 19
Chapter 7: Week Six 22
Chapter 8: Week Seven 26
Chapter 9: Week Eight 30
Chapter 10: Week Nine 33

BOOK 4

Introduction 37
Chapter 1: Vegetarian Breakfast Recipes 39
Chapter 2: Vegetarian Lunch Recipes 44
Chapter 3: Vegetarian Dinner Recipes 50
Chapter 4: Vegetarian Smoothie, Shakes and Juice Recipes 58
Chapter 5: Vegetarian Dessert Recipes 66

Book 3

Chapter 1: Sweets And Snack Options

In this chapter you will be introduced to some great Vegetarian snacks. These snack options range from sweet to savoury, so there is something for whatever you are craving. Many of these snack options also allow room for you to add your own twist. You can add different fruits, vegetables or seasonings to make them more appealing to you.

Vegan 'Yogurt'

Ingredients:

- Coconut milk- 28 ounces
- Agar Agar- 1-tablespoon
- Sugar Or Maple Syrup- 2 tablespoons
- Probiotic Capsules- 4

Instructions:

Add shaken coconut milk to a pan. Whisk smooth. Sprinkle Agar Agar onto the coconut milk. Simmer this mix. Turn the heat to low, and cook 10 minutes, whisking occasionally, until the Agar Agar has completely dissolved.

Cool until this is just warm to the touch. Add the ingredients from 4 probiotic capsules. Whisk and taste.

Add up sugar or maple syrup.

Pour the yogurt into canning jars fresh from the dishwasher. Using fresh lids, cap each jar, and place in the oven for 24 hours with the light on for warmth. Do not disturb! Chill the yogurt for 6 hours, checking to make sure it has not separated. If so, stir well, and use that jar first.

Greek Style Quick Yogurt

Ingredients:

- Coconut Meat- 2 cups
- Coconut Water- ½ cup
- Probiotic Capsules- 4
- Pink sea salt- just a bit
- Feel free to add Carrots, Apples, Bananas, or any other small fruit of your choosing

Instructions:

Blend 2 cups young coconut meat, ½ cup coconut water, the ingredients from 4 probiotic capsules, and a bit of pink sea salt. Blend, starting on low, and slowly increasing, until the mixture is super-smooth. Sweeten to taste. Place in container and refrigerate at least two hours.

Chips And Salsa
Ingredients:

- Large Beefsteak Tomatoes- 4
- Jalapeno- ½
- Scallions- 3
- Cilantro- a handful

Instructions:

Coarse chop 4 large beefsteak tomatoes. Mix ½ jalapeno (seeded and chopped), 3 scallions and a handful of cilantro in a bowl. Layer these, or add in garlic, pineapple, watermelon, zucchini, green pepper, strawberries, or what you enjoy. Serve with pita, corn, or tofu chips.

Toast With Fruit Butter

Ingredients:

- Seasonal Fruit
- Sugar- 1 cup per pint of fruit
- Fruit Pectin- 1 package per 4 pints of fruit
- Lemon Juice
- Spices of your choice

Instructions:

Place three small plates in the freezer. Using your slow cooker, take seasonal fruit, a bit of sugar (1 cup per pint), fruit pectin (one packet for every 4 pints), and lemon juice; plus any spices that you would enjoy. On low, stir at 1 hour, then at the 2-hour mark. Cover, raise to high, and cook 2-3 hours. Test a spoonful of jam by seeing if it becomes firm on a plate from the freezer. If not, cook a while longer.

Muffin Square

Ingredients:

- Ripe Bananas- 2 large
- Vanilla- 1 tsp (optional)
- Rolled Oats- 2 cups
- Salt- ½ tsp (optional)
- Dried Dates- ¼ cup
- Chopped Nuts- ¼ cup

Instructions:

Peel and mash 2 large, very ripe bananas, until there are no large chunks left. Add 1 teaspoon vanilla (optional), 2 cups rolled oats, 1/2 teaspoon salt (optional), 1/4 cup pitted, chopped dried dates, and 1/4 cup chopped nuts — such as walnuts, hazelnuts, or pecans, stirring well after each addition.

Pat into a well-oiled 9 x 9 pan, and bake in a 350 degree oven for 30 minutes, or until the edges begin to crisp. Place the pan on a wire rack, and cut into bars when mostly cool.

Chapter 2: Week One

Day 1:

Breakfast: Mango/orange/beet juice smoothie

Noon Meal: Southwest Salad-greens with black beans, corn and peppers

Evening Meal: Sun-dried tomatoes, Spinach, and Tofu <u>Quiche</u> (save some for later)

Sun-Dried Tomatoes, Spinach, And Tofu <u>Quiche</u>

Ingredients:

- Ground Flax
- Water
- Almond Flour
- Dried Parsley
- Dried Oregano
- Kosher Salt
- Drained Tofu
- Garlic Cloves
- Mushrooms
- Fresh Chives
- Basil Leaves
- Sun-Dried Tomatoes
- Baby Spinach
- Nutritional Yeast
- Sea Salt
- Black And Rep Pepper

Instructions:

Whisk 1 tablespoon ground flax and 3 tablespoons water. Set aside to let gel.

Stir together 1 cup almond flour, 1 cup oat flour, 1 teaspoon dried parsley, 1 teaspoon dried oregano, and 1/2 tsp. kosher salt. Add the gelled flax mixture, and some water (no more than 3 tablespoons) until it is stick together when pressed between your fingers.

Working from the centre, press into a crust to the top of the rim of an oiled pan. Poke a few holes with a fork so air can escape, and bake at 350 degrees for 13-15 minutes.

Meanwhile, break apart and blend 14 ounces pressed and drained tofu until creamy. Add a bit of almond mix if needed. In a skillet, sauté 1 thin sliced leek and 3 minced garlic cloves. Once tender add 8-oz sliced mushrooms, and cook until most of the moisture is go- about 10 minutes. Add 1/2 cup chopped fresh chives, 1/2 cup chopped fresh basil leaves, 1/3 cup chopped oil-packed sun-dried tomatoes, 1-cup baby spinach, 2 tbsp. nutritional yeast, 1 teaspoon dried oregano, 3/4-1 teaspoon fine grain sea salt. And black and rep pepper, to taste, Cook until the spinach is completely wilted.

Remove from heat, and add the tofu mixture. Stir until completely combined. Spoon into baked crust, and bake at 375 degrees for 30-40 minutes, until the top of the quiche is done. Cool 20 minutes on a baking rack for the easiest cutting.

Day 2:

Breakfast: Oats or other cereal and fruit

Noon Meal: Fresh spring mix with leftovers from last night

Evening Meal: Baked Ziti with vegetables

Day 3:

Breakfast: Overnight oats with fresh or canned fruits

Noon Meal: Tostada

Tostadas

Ingredients:

- Corn Tortillas
- Broth
- Chopped Onion
- Minced Garlic
- Black Beans
- Lemon
- Cumin
- Green Chillies
- Salt And Pepper

Instructions:

Toast 8 good-quality corn tortillas in the oven, or individually in a pan, until brown and crunchy.

Heat 3 tablespoons broth, or 1 tablespoon oil, and sauté 1 medium chopped onion and 2 cloves minced garlic about 5 minutes, or until golden. Add ¼ cup water, 2 15 cans of drained, rinsed black beans (use your own if you have them), the juice of ½ lemon, 2 teaspoons cumin, and 2 small seeded and sliced hot green chillies (optional). Salt and pepper to taste. Mash, and remove from heat.

Spread tortillas with a generous serving of the bean mixture, and top with greens, tomatoes, corn, avocados, cashew cream, and salsa.

<u>Evening Meal: Quiche, and a fresh salad</u>

Day 4:

Breakfast: Fresh fruit

Noon Meal: Creamy soup- tomato, cauliflower, or mushroom

Evening Meal: Mexican Black Bean 'Pizza'

Day 5:

Breakfast: Cereal with peaches, cinnamon, and walnuts

Noon Meal: Quiche from Day 2

Evening Meal: Hearty Roasted Vegetables

Hearty Roasted Vegetables

Ingredients:

- Brussels Sprouts
- Cauliflower
- Hard-Shell Squash
- Button Mushrooms
- Small Onions
- Honey-Balsamic Vinegar-Garlic Mix
- Salt And Pepper

Instructions:
Start with 8 oz. of Brussels sprouts, halved. Keeping this as an average size, break apart 1 cauliflower, and cut up 2 hard-shell squash (acorn is a good choice) into cubes about the same size. Add 12 oz. button mushrooms and two small onions quartered. Mix well, and place on lined cookie sheets. Bake at 350 degrees for 20 to 30 minutes, turning once halfway through. Baste the vegetables with a honey-balsamic vinegar-garlic mix, and season with salt and pepper and other spices if desired. Roast 5 more minutes, turn once again, and baste the vegetables again.

Chapter 3: Week Two

Day 1:

Breakfast: Muffin Squares

Noon Meal: Southwest Wrap of tofu, leftover pasta bake or chickpeas; spring mix; and a spicy dressing in a whole-wheat tortilla

Evening Meal: Pasta and Portobello mushrooms with extra soup or vodka sauce

Day 2:

Breakfast: Jelly-filled muffins

Jelly-Filled Muffins

Ingredients:

- All-Purpose Flour
- Baking Powder
- Baking Soda
- Ground Nutmeg
- Fine Salt
- Soy Or Rice Milk
- Granulated Sugar
- Vegetable Oil
- Vanilla Extract
- Muffin Cups With Paper Liners

Instructions:

In a large bowl, sift together 1 1/2 cups all-purpose flour, 3/4-teaspoon baking powder, 1/2-teaspoon baking soda, 1/2-teaspoon ground nutmeg, 1/2-teaspoon fine salt. Set aside.

In a glass or plastic bowl, mix 1-cup plain soy or rice milk, 1-teaspoon cider vinegar, and 2 tablespoons cornstarch. Mix until the cornstarch has dissolved. Make a well in the dry ingredients, and pour the milk mixture into the well. Stir well, adding 3/4 cup plus 2 tablespoons granulated sugar, 1/3-cup vegetable oil, and 2 teaspoons vanilla extract. There will be a few lumps in the mixture.

Line the full-sized muffin cups with paper liners, and fill each one about ¾ full. Using a spoon, put a small indentation in the batter, and fills each with 1 heaping teaspoon of raspberry, strawberry, or grape jam or preserves. Bake in a 350-degree oven for about 20-25 minutes, until the tops of the muffins are firm. Remove from pan, and cool completely on a wire rack.

Noon Meal: Vegan Mac and cheese- add fruit salad for a full meal

Evening Meal: Three-bean chilli and Pesto

Day 3:

Breakfast: Cereal and fruit

Noon Meal: Wrap Day: rice, beans and greens

Evening Meal: Shepard's pie- make extra of the vegetable stew to use for lunch

Day 4:

Breakfast: Apple/peach/kale smoothie

Noon Meal: Vegetable stew

Evening Meal: Baked Lasagna Rolls

Baked Lasagna Rolls

Ingredients:

- Eggplants
- Salt
- Whole-Wheat Lasagna Noodles
- Tofu 'Cheese'
- Tomato Sauce

Instructions:

Slice 2 eggplants into ¼ inch strips lengthwise, salt and place in a colander in the sink to drain and shed bitterness. Then rinse, place on kitchen towel, and use a weighted cookie sheet to remove excess water. Then bake for 13-15 minutes in a 425-degree oven, turning oven down to 375 once eggplant is done. Set aside or use cooked whole-wheat lasagna noodles.

Make the tofu 'cheese': 2 lemons, juiced (~1/3 cup), 1 12-ounce block extra firm tofu, drained and pressed dry for 10 minutes. 3 Tbsp. nutritional yeast, 1/2 cup fresh basil, finely chopped, 1 Tbsp. dried oregano, 3-4 Tbsp. extra virgin olive oil, and salt and pepper to taste. Pulse in a food processor or blender, scraping when needed, until there are only small bits of basil showing.

Pour tomato sauce into the bottom of a baking dish, reserving some for topping. Scoop a generous amount of the tofu cheese mixture onto the slices/noodles, and roll up. Place each roll seam-side down in the tomato sauce. Add additional sauce on top of the rolls if wished. Bake 15-30 minutes, until the rolls are lightly browned.

Day 5:

Breakfast: Fruit salad

Noon Meal: Pita Pizzas

Evening Meal: Tangiers of apricots, couscous and chickpeas

Tangiers Of Apricots, Couscous And Chickpeas

Less a recipe than a cooking style, this is a method of a loosely covered pot, with all the ingredients cooking down and absorbing the flavours of the stock and each other.

Chapter 4: Week Three

Day 1:

Breakfast: Citrus-Granola Parfait

Citrus-Granola Parfait

Ingredients:

- Nuts
- Dried Coconut
- Zests Of A Lemon
- Orange
- Maple Syrup
- Vanilla Extract
- Top Soy Or Other Yogurts
- Cereal

Instructions:

Use seeds, nuts, dried coconut, plus the zests of a lemon, a lime, and an orange. Use the juices, some maple syrup, and vanilla extract to the mix, and stir in oats. Blend well, and dry in a 300-degree oven for 15 minutes, stir, and bake another 15 minutes. Cool completely, and use to top soy or other yogurts, or add a bit of unexpected crunch to your morning cereal.

Noon Meal: Vegan Sushi rolls- a great calcium boost!

Evening Meal: Portobello Marsala

Day 2:

Breakfast: Oats with almond milk and fresh fruit

Noon Meal: White Bean and Avocado Club sandwich

White Bean And Avocado Club Sandwich

Ingredients:

- Bread
- White Bean Paste
- Leaf Lettuce, Or Basil Leaves
- Avocado Slices
- Onion

Instructions:

Using your favourite bread, spread white bean paste on one, top with a second slice of bread, or leaf lettuce, or basil leaves. Add avocado slices, onion, or other topping, and top with bread. Bring lots of napkins!

Evening Meal: Quiche with Chard and chickpeas

Day 3:

Breakfast: Jelly-filled Muffins

Noon Meal: Pasta and pesto

Evening Meal: Peanut-Squash Stew and a fresh salad

Day 4:

Breakfast: Breakfast Toast

Breakfast Toast

This is simple, and quick. Toast your favorite bread, and spread it with refried beans. Top with avocados and onions; greens, tomatoes, and seeds, or any other combination that your taste buds enjoy!

Noon Meal: Twice-Baked Potato Boats

Twice-Baked Potato Boats

Ingredients:

- Potatoes
- Vegan Sour Cream
- Corn
- Black Bean
- Pinto Beans
- Celery
- Vegan Cheese

Instructions:

Bake 6 potatoes at 350 degrees until soft. Remove from oven and cool. Scoop out the potato flesh, leaving about a ¼ inch all around for stability. Place the scooped potatoes into a pan, and add a small amount of stock and continue cooking them. Mash well.

Stir in vegan sour cream, corn, black bean, pinto beans, celery, vegan cheese, or other toppings. Refill potato boats, heaping a bit. Return to the oven, and bake until topping is golden brown, about 15-20 minutes.

Evening Meal: Eggplant with tomatoes and basil

Day 5:

Breakfast: Cereal and fresh/frozen fruit

Noon Meal: Jackfruit in BBQ sauce, on rolls

Evening Meal: Texas-style 'Chilli' (use eggplant instead of meat), salad with leafy greens and avocado-cilantro dressing.

Chapter 5: Week Four

Day 1:

Breakfast: Muffin Squares

Noon Meal: Pita salad with dressing

Evening Meal: Potato Gnocchi With Vodka Sauce

Potato Gnocchi With Vodka Sauce

Ingredients:

- Mashed Potato
- Salt And Pepper
- Flour

Instructions:

Mix left-over mashed potato (the drier the better) or the flesh of two or three baked potatoes, mashed without milk or butter, a bit of salt and pepper and a few tablespoons of flour. Turn onto a board, and knead. The more you work this, the more flour you will require from the moisture of the potatoes. Work until this is dry enough to separate into 4 sections, and form a long roll from each section.

Use a sharp knife to cut these into pieces, and roll them individually in flour. If the touch, they are likely to stick together.

Bring a large pan of water or stock to a boil, and drop a few of these in at a time. They will sink, and then rise to the surface when they are done. Remove and toss with a small amount of oil to stop them from sticking together. Serve with sauce, and enjoy.

Day 2:

Breakfast: overnight oats

Noon Meal: Beans and Greens

Beans And Greens

Ingredients:

- Vegetable Broth
- Onion
- Bell Pepper
- Black Beans
- Rice
- Soy Sauce

- Swiss Chard
- Tomato Sauce
- Red Chilli Powder
- Nutritional Yeast
- Salt
- Ground Seeds

Instructions:
In a large pan with a tight-fitting lid, warm the vegetable broth, then add onion and bell pepper. Once these are tender, add 1-cup pre-cooked black beans, ½ cup pre-cooked rice, and 2 tablespoons soy sauce. Once these are warm, lower the heat, and add 3-4 cups Swiss chard or other greens, and cover tightly until the greens have wilted. Once the wilting is complete, add tomato sauce, a dash of red chilli powder, nutritional yeast, and salt to taste. Top with 1-2 tablespoons ground seeds, and completely warm before serving.

Evening Meal: Taco Bowls with Tempeh

Day 3:

Breakfast: Smoothie

Noon Meal: Risotto Cakes with marina

Evening Meal: Asparagus and Lemon Risotto (fry extra in cakes for lunch)

Asparagus And Lemon Risotto

Ingredients:
- Asparagus
- Vegetable Stock
- Olive Oil
- Rice
- Lemon
- Tarragon

Instructions:
Blanch 6 stalks of asparagus for 2 minutes: it will be crunchy. Set in ice water until cool. Take the tips off, and either shaves the stalks for garnish or save for use later. If you use canned asparagus, skip this step.

Warm 1-quart vegetable stock, and in a separate, deep pan, warm ta bit of olive oil, and coat 1 cup of rice until it is evenly shiny. Add about 1/3 of a cup of the stock at a time to the rice until the stock is gone, stirring constantly to avoid burning or sticking.

Set aside any extra you may have made, and add the juice of 2 lemons and the asparagus tips. Taste, and season with tarragon.

Day 4:

Breakfast: Cereal with almond milk and fruit

Noon Meal: Wheat-protein "French Dip"

Wheat-Protein "French Dip"

Cut Seitan into strips, and fry in oil. Place on a crusty roll. Serve with vegetable stock -adding a drop of liquid smoke for flavor- and Dijon-style mustard.

Evening Meal: Seven-layer Pie

Day 5:

Breakfast: Jelly Muffin

Noon Meal: Hard-shell squash with apples, meat substitute, and bread cubes

Evening Meal: One-pot Meal with Pasta

One-Pot Meal With Pasta

This recipe uses pasta, vegetables, greens, and sauces to ease cooking times. For the south-western version of this dish, use corn (fire roasted if you have it in season), cilantro, black and pinto beans, fresh onion, chili powder, cumin and pasta to make a quick, simple dish.

Chapter 6: Week Five

Day 1:

Breakfast: Overnight oats with tropical fruits

Noon Meal: Hummus, carrots and celery

Evening Meal: Cauliflower-rice stir-fry

Day 2:

Breakfast: Lentils and onions in a tomato sauce- a traditional breakfast

Noon Meal: Steamed vegetables with Garlic sauce

Steamed Vegetables With Garlic Sauce

Ingredients:

- Garlic Cloves
- Shallots
- Sea Salt
- Black Pepper
- Cornstarch
- Vegetable Stock

Instructions:

Sauté 8 garlic cloves and 2 shallots in olive oil, seasoning with a touch of sea salt and black pepper. Cook until soft. Very slowly, add up to 4 teaspoons cornstarch, then 1-cup vegetable stock, whisking well between additions to avoid lumps.

Evening Meal: Pineapple and Cashews, stir-fried

Day 3:

Breakfast: Quinoa, apple and carrot porridge

Noon Meal: Wheat berry Salad

Wheat Berry Salad

Ingredients:

- Wheat Berries
- Pan-Toast Nuts
- Celery
- Dried Fruits
- Herbs
- Lemon Juice

- Olive Oil
- Salt
- Pepper

Instructions:

Cook 1 ½ cups hard wheat berries in enough water to cover for about an hour, set aside. Pan-toast nuts, and add them to celery, dried fruits, and herbs. Once the wheat berries are cool, add them to the other ingredients. Taste and add lemon juice, olive oil, salt, or fresh pepper as desired.

Evening Meal: Spring mix topped with shredded Carrot and Avocado

Day 4:

Breakfast: Vegetable-based smoothie

Noon Meal: Orange-ginger Tofu with broccoli

Evening Meal: Mushroom Brown Rice with ginger

Day 5:

Breakfast: Lemon-Baked Tofu With Vegan Yogurt

Lemon-Baked Tofu With Vegan Yogurt

Ingredients:

- Extra Firm Tofu
- Lemon Juice
- Balsamic Vinegar
- Soy Sauce
- Lemon Zest
- Olive Oil

Instructions:

Slice 1 lb. extra firm tofu (drained and pressed) that has been sliced into ½ inch slices, and pour over a marinate of 5 tablespoons lemon juice, 1 teaspoon balsamic vinegar, 1 tablespoon soy sauce, 1teaspoon lemon zest, and 1 tablespoon olive oil that has been mixed well. Let marinate for 30 minutes, turning once. Bake 20-30 minutes at 350 degrees.

Noon Meal: Mushroom Stroganoff

Evening Meal: Coconut-Vegetable Rice

Coconut-Vegetable Rice

Ingredients:

- Jasmine Rice
- Coconut Milk
- Cilantro
- Lime Juice
- Mushrooms
- Olive Oil
- Zucchini
- Red Pepper
- Minced Garlic
- Fresh Ginger
- Frozen Edamame
- Scallions Sliced

Instructions:

Steam 1 cup jasmine rice in a rice cooker with ¾ cup of coconut milk and 1 ¼ water. When complete, add 1-cup cilantro and the juice of 2 limes.

While cooking, in a large pan, sauté 8 oz. sliced mushrooms in 2 tablespoons olive oil until tender, Add 2 small sliced zucchini, 1 diced red pepper, 2 cloves minced garlic, and a tablespoon of fresh ginger. Cook for another minute.

Add to this a bit more coconut milk, ½ c frozen edamame, and 2 scallions sliced. Season to taste, and serve over the jasmine rice.

Chapter 7: Week Six

Day 1:
Breakfast: Breakfast toast

Noon Meal: Steam sugar snap peas and carrots, toss with balsamic and noodles

Evening Meal: Butternut Squash tortellini with pesto

Day 2:
Breakfast: Peach/orange smoothie

Noon Meal: Black-Bean Burger

Evening Meal: **Ratatouille**

Ingredients:

- Bell Peppers
- Soy Sauce
- Balsamic Vinegar
- Agave Nectar
- Japanese Eggplants
- Yellow Squash
- Zucchini
- Onion
- Tomatoes
- Garlic

Instructions:

Place bell peppers (red or yellow for color) onto a foil-lined cookie sheet and broil turning every 3-5 minutes until there is char on all sides. Place the peppers in a bowl and cover with plastic wrap for 5 minutes. Meanwhile, mix 2 tablespoons soy sauce, 2 tablespoons balsamic vinegar, and 2 tablespoons agave nectar in a bowl or gallon bag, mixing well. Turn down the oven to 400 degrees.

Cut 2 small Japanese eggplants, 2 small yellow squash, 1 small zucchini into ¼ to ½ inch cubes. Cut a small onion into eights, and add all the vegetables to the marinate, tossing lightly. Let the marinate rest for at least 5 minutes. Peel the skin, seeds and stems from the bell peppers, reserving any juice. Dice the peppers into ½ inch cubes, and place in the bowl with the reserved juices.

Cut 4 tomatoes in half horizontally, and scoop out most of the seeds with a knife or small spoon. Place on a parchment covered baking sheet. Place a garlic clove into the seed cavity of each tomato so the garlic does not burn.

Sprinkle lightly with rosemary. Spread the vegetables from the marinate onto the rest of the sheet, and bake for 30 minutes, turning the cubed vegetables halfway through. Baste with the remaining marinate if they look dry.

Set the cubed vegetable into the bowl with the peppers, and place the tomato halves into a pan. The skins should slide off, once they are removed, mash the tomato flesh and the garlic. Once the tomatoes have reduced, add to the other vegetables, and serve over rice or pasta.

Day 3:

Breakfast: Baked Doughnuts With Fruit

Baked Doughnuts With Fruit

Ingredients:

- Vegan Sugar
- Unsweetened Applesauce
- Plant Milk
- Grape Seed Oil
- Vanilla
- Flour
- Baking Powder
- Baking Soda
- Fresh Fruit

Instructions:

In a large bowl, mix ½ c vegan sugar, ½ c unsweetened applesauce, 1 c plant milk, plus 1 tablespoon, 2 tablespoons grape seed oil and 2 teaspoons vanilla until well-blended. Gradually, add 2 cups flour, 1-teaspoon baking powder and ½ teaspoon of baking soda, and ½ teaspoon total of spices that blend with your fruit. Gently fold in 1-cup fresh fruit.

Oil the doughnut pan, and fill each section about ¾ full. Bake at 325 for about 15 minutes, or until the tops brown. Cool completely before removing from the pan.

Noon Meal: Pita "Gyros", tofu or tempeh instead of meat

Evening Meal: Chickpea tempura-coated vegetables

Day 4:
Breakfast: Cereal with fresh fruit

Noon Meal: Fruit salad on greens

Evening Meal: Roasted sweet potatoes with pinto/black bean burritos

Roasted Sweet Potatoes With Pinto/Black Bean Burritos
Ingredients:

- Sweet Potatoes
- Chickpeas
- Olive Oil
- Cumin
- Coriander
- Cinnamon
- Smoked (Or Regular) Paprika
- Salt Or Lemon Juice
- Sauce Of Hummus
- Garlic And Spices

Instructions:

Scrub and halve 4 medium sweet potatoes.

In a bowl, mix a15-ounce can chickpeas, 1/2 Tbsp. olive oil, and 1/2 tsp. each cumin, coriander, cinnamon, smoked (or regular) paprika. Taste, and a bit of salt or lemon juice if needed.

Place the sweet potatoes cut-side down on a foil-lined baking dish. Add the chickpea mixture, and bake at 400 degrees for about 20-25 minutes, or until tender.

Make a simple sauce of hummus, lemon juice, garlic and spices to top these.

Day 5:
Breakfast: Chocolate Nut Butter on toast

Noon Meal: Pot Pie

Evening Meal: Greek-style Caponata

Greek-Style Caponata

Ingredients:

- Diced Tomatoes
- Zucchini
- Summer Squash
- Tomatoes Cut Into Wedges
- Large Japanese Eggplant
- Red Onion
- Potato
- Minced Garlic
- Olive Oil
- Salt
- Pepper And Oregano

Instructions:

Into a casserole dish, pour 1 14 or 15 ounce can of diced tomatoes and their juices, and spread to cover the bottom of the pan. In a bowl, combine 2 sliced zucchini, 2 summer squash, 2 tomatoes cut into wedges, a large Japanese eggplant, cut into 1 inch rounds, a red onion cut into wedges, 1 potato, cut into 1 inch cubes, 3 cloves of minced garlic, ¼ cup olive oil, and salt, pepper and oregano to taste. Pour the vegetable mixture over the tomatoes, and bake in a 400 degree oven for 30 minutes covered with foil, then about 40 minutes uncovered, or until the vegetables are golden.

Chapter 8: Week Seven

Day 1:

Breakfast: Chickpea Pancake With Seasonal Fruits

Chickpea Pancake With Seasonal Fruits

Ingredients:

- Green Onion
- Bell Peppers
- Chickpea Flour
- Garlic Powder
- Finely Ground Sea Salt
- Finely Ground Black Pepper
- Baking Powder
- Red Pepper Flakes
  Mushrooms, Cashew Cream, Avocados, Hummus Or Salsa
- For Topping

Instructions:

Finely chop 1 green onion, ¼ cup bell peppers. Mix ½ cup chickpea flour, ¼ garlic powder, ¼ teaspoon finely ground sea salt, 1/8 teaspoon finely ground black pepper, and ¼ teaspoon baking powder. Add a pinch of red pepper flakes if you wish. Mix well, adding in ½ cup water- a bit more may be needed.

In a well-oiled pan, pour one or two pancakes. These cook more slowly than traditional pancakes, and need spread out. Turn when you can slide a spatula completely under the pancake. Cook for a similar amount of time on the other side. Top with mushrooms, cashew cream, avocados, hummus or salsa.

Noon Meal: Rice Noodles and vegetables, garnished with mandarin oranges

Evening Meal: Baked Spaghetti Squash with fresh pepper, oil and vegan cheese

Day 2:

Breakfast: Baked Doughnuts

Noon Meal: Steamed Tofu-Vegetable Pot Stickers With Peanut Sauce

Steamed Tofu-Vegetable Pot Stickers With Peanut Sauce

Ingredients:

- Minced Garlic Clove
- Fresh Ginger
- Pressed Tofu
- Chopped Scallion
- Tofu Mixture

Instructions:

In a skillet, sauté 1 minced garlic clove and ½ teaspoon fresh ginger for about a minute. Crumble and sauté 8 ounces drained and pressed tofu for about 5 minutes more. Add one chopped scallion, and remove from heat.

Place the won ton wrapper in a diamond shape in front of you. Put 1 teaspoon of the tofu mixture in the center of the wrapper and moisten the upper diamond edges. Fold the bottom up, then each side in to meet the bottom corner (looks like an envelope). Fold the top down, and seal with the edges. Place seam side down in a bamboo steamer. Leave room between these! Steam for 5 minutes until the outer surface is shiny and a few bubbles form.

Evening Meal: Chard and Chickpea with pasta

Day 3:

Breakfast: Jelly Muffins

Noon Meal: Portobello 'burgers' with all the trimmings

Evening Meal: Pine Nut Sauce On Rice

Pine Nut Sauce On Rice

Ingredients:

- Grape Or Cherry Tomatoes
- Kalamata Olives
- Minced Garlic Cloves

- Olive Oil
- Fresh Lemon Juice
- Balsamic Vinegar
- Sea Salt
- Black Pepper
- Pine Nuts
- Fresh Basil

Instructions:

Halve 2 1/2 cups grape or cherry tomatoes, and place in a giant bowl. Add 1/2 cup kalamata olives, pitted and chopped, 5 large minced garlic cloves, 1/4 cup olive oil, 2 tablespoons fresh lemon juice, 1 tablespoon balsamic vinegar, 2 teaspoons sea salt (taste first!), freshly ground black pepper (to taste), and mix well. Toast 1/4 cup pine nuts in a dry pan on medium-low heat, shaking often this should take less than 5 minutes. Place the tomato mixture in a serving dish, and top with the pine nuts and 1/2 cup chopped fresh basil.

Day 4:

Breakfast: Oatmeal/porridge with fruits

Noon Meal: Winter Lentil Soup

Evening Meal: Stuffed Green Peppers

Stuffed Green Peppers

Ingredients:

- Cooked Brown Rice
- Small Tomatoes
- Frozen Corn
- Sweet Onion
- Ripe Olives
- Canned Black Beans
- Canned Red Beans
- Fresh Basil Leaves
- Garlic Cloves
- Salt
- Pepper
- Vegan Cheese
- Spaghetti Sauce

Instructions:

Combine 2 cups cooked brown rice, 3 small tomatoes, chopped, 1 cup frozen corn, thawed, 1 small sweet onion, chopped, 1 can (4-1/4 ounces) chopped ripe olives, 1/3 cup canned black beans, rinsed and drained, 1/3 cup canned red beans, rinsed and drained, 4 fresh basil leaves, thinly sliced, 3 garlic cloves, minced, 1 teaspoon salt, and 1/2 teaspoon pepper. Add ¾ cup vegan cheese, if desired.

Cut the tops off of 6 large sweet peppers, and remove the seeds, being careful not to break the pepper. Fill each pepper with the rice mixture, and place in a crock pot Cover the bottom of the pot and the peppers with 3/4 cup spaghetti sauce and 1/2 cup water. Cook for 3 ½ to 4 hours on low.

Day 5:

Breakfast: Blueberry/Banana Smoothie- a bit of orange adds zest!

Noon Meal: Sloppy Joe's- with red or brown lentils instead of meat

Evening Meal: Slow-Cooker Jambalaya

Chapter 9: Week Eight

Day 1:

Breakfast: Cereal with ginger, apple, and agave

Noon Meal: Black Bean Quesadillas

Evening Meal: Italian-Inspired Soup

Italian-Inspired Soup

Ingredients:

- Olive Oil
- White Onion
- Carrots
- Celery
- Cloves Garlic
- Vegetable Stock
- Fire-Roasted Tomatoes
- Wheat Pasta
- Dried Thyme
- Dried Oregano
- Rosemary
- Spinach

Instructions:

In a stockpot, heat 2 tablespoons olive oil, and sauté one small white onion until tender. Add 1-cup carrots, cut into rounds, 1-cup celery cut into similar sized pieces, and 3 cloves garlic. Sauté for an additional 3 minutes.

Add 6 cups vegetable stock, a 14 ounce can fire-roasted tomatoes, 8 ounces whole-wheat pasta (orzo is a good choice), 1/2 teaspoon dried thyme, ¼ teaspoon dried oregano and 1/4 teaspoon rosemary, and stir to combine well. After about 10 minutes, add 4 cups spinach. Cook until the spinach is wilted, and test pasta to insure it is done.

Day 2:

Breakfast: Green Smoothie

Green Smoothie

Blend 1-cup berries, 1 handful of greens, a small banana, and orange juice until smooth- adding either water or juice to thin if needed.

Noon Meal: Broccoli and white bean soup- creamy or chunky!

Evening Meal: Vegan pizza

Day 3:

Breakfast: Walnut and spice stuffed apples (make extra to freeze)

Noon Meal: Peanut noodles

Evening Meal: Red Pepper And Pinto Frittata

Red Pepper And Pinto Frittata
Ingredients:

- Pinto Beans
- Red Pepper
- Sweet Onion
- Carrot
- Garlic
- Broccoli
- Plum Tomato
- Chickpea Flour
- Vegetable Stock
- Dried Basil
- Black Salt
- Nutritional Yeast

Instructions:

Pre-cook 1 cup Pinto Beans, drained and rinsed, 1-cup red pepper, chopped, 1 cup sweet onion, chopped, 1/2 cup carrot, grated, 2 tbsp. garlic, minced, 1/2 cup broccoli, divided into mini florets, and 1 plum tomato, diced. These can be left overs. Heat the oven to 400 degrees, and oil a cake pan.

In a small bowl, mix 1-cup chickpea flour with 1-cup water until it is a smooth paste. Bring 1 ½ cups vegetable stock, 1 tablespoon dried basil, ½ teaspoon black salt, and 3 tablespoons nutritional yeast to a boil. Add the chickpea flour mixture, and reduce the heat. Stir constantly until the batter thickens, and cook for another 3 minutes afterwards.

Add the bean and red pepper mixture, folding it in gently. Pour into the oil pan, and bake for 25-30 minutes. Let cool before removing from pan.

Day 4:

Breakfast: Breakfast parfait

Noon Meal: Twice-baked potato boats

Evening Meal: Cucumbers, avocados, and onions in a slightly spicy Asian dressing

Day 5:

Breakfast: Cherry Dumplings

Cherry Dumplings

Ingredients:

- Cherries
- Flour
- Baking Powder
- Sugar
- Vegan Margarine
- Plant Milk

Instructions:

In a deep pan, bring to a gentle boil 2 cups cherries, and 1 cup water, adjusting the sweetness for your taste- they should be just slightly sour to balance the dumpling.

Stir together 2 cups flour, 2 teaspoons baking powder, ½ teaspoon sugar, 2 tablespoons vegan margarine, and ¾ cup plant milk. Scoop out with a teaspoon, and gently drop the dumplings into the pot one at a time, making sure that they are completely covered. Steam with the lid on loosely for 10-15 minutes. Break open the largest of the dumplings, and make sure they are fluffy all the way through. Serve hot, or remove the cherries and store the dumpling separately for later enjoyment. **Noon Meal:** Quinoa with edamame and corn **Evening Meal:** Seven-vegetable couscous

Chapter 10: Week Nine

Day 1:

Breakfast: Tofu Breakfast Scramble

Tofu Breakfast Scramble

Cook 4 ounces of drained tofu and 2 spring onions (or one leek) in a pan with a bit of oil for one minute; add 2 teaspoons tamari, 2 tablespoons savory yeast flakes, ½ teaspoon turmeric, and 2 to 3 tablespoons water and cook for another minute. Serve with toast, has browns, or English muffin,

Noon Meal: Vegetable stew

Evening Meal: Vegan Alfredo With Peas And Kale

Vegan Alfredo With Peas And Kale

Ingredients:

- Minced Garlic Cloves
- Arrowroot Powder
- Plant Milk
- Salt And Pepper
- Nutritional Yeast
- Garlic Powder
- Vegan Parmesan

Instructions:

Sauté 4 minced garlic cloves in oil until tender. Add 4 tablespoons arrowroot powder, and whisk until smooth. Add ¼ cup at a time 1 ¾ cup plant milk, whisking well to avoid lumps. Cook for 2 minutes.

Transfer to a blender, and salt and pepper to taste. Add 4 tablespoons nutritional yeast, and ½ teaspoon garlic powder. Blend on high until creamy. Up to ¼ cup of vegan Parmesan may be added, as well.

Return to pan, and cook on medium heat until it bubbles, then turn the heat to low and continue to cook until it thickens. You may need to add an additional ¼ cup of plant milk, or remove ½ cup of the sauce, and add 1-teaspoon arrowroot whisked well, to thicken more.

Serve over pasta, and top with fresh vegetables.

Day 2:
Breakfast: Jelly Muffin

Noon Meal: Mushroom Pho

Evening Meal: Asparagus and Carrot Indian Stir Fry

Day 3:
Breakfast: Muffin Square

Noon Meal: BLT- sprouts, avocado, fresh basil, tomatoes, and vegan bacon

Evening Meal: Chard, chickpea, and rice casserole

Day 4:

Breakfast: Lemon Scones

Lemon Scones
Ingredients:

- All-Purpose Flour
- Sugar
- Baking Powder
- Baking Soda
- Salt
- Lemon Zest
- Cold Coconut Oil
- Almond Milk
- Lemon Juice
- Apple Cider Vinegar
- Vanilla Extract

Instructions:

Mix together in a large bowl 3 1/4 cup all-purpose flour, 1/2-cup sugar, 1 T baking powder, 1/2 t baking soda, 1 t salt and 2 T lemon zest. Using a pastry cutter or a fork cut in 8 T cold coconut oil until the mixture is evenly crumbly.

In a small bowl, mix 1 1/2 cups almond milk, 1/3 cup lemon juice, and 1 T apple cider vinegar. Let sit for 2 minutes or until the milk begins to curdle. Add 1 t vanilla extract, and pour the liquids into the dry ingredients and mix well. Dough will be sticky, so knead it a few times, and pat into a circle about 2 inches thick on a parchment paper-covered cookie sheet. Brush with almond milk and sprinkle with sugar. Bake in a 400-degree oven for 20 to 25 minutes or until golden brown.

Noon Meal: Chick-less noodle soup

Evening Meal: Vegan Pizza

Day 5:

Breakfast: Strawberry pancakes

Strawberry Pancakes

Ingredients:

- Flour
- Rolled Oats
- Baking Powder
- Salt
- Pure Vanilla Extract
- Sugar
- Plant Milk
- Unrefined Coconut Oil
- Chopped Strawberries
- Fruit Butter

Instructions:

Combine 1/3-cup flour, 2 tbsp. rolled oats, 2/3 tsp. baking powder, and 1/8 tsp. salt. Add 1/2 tsp. pure vanilla extract, 1 tbsp. sugar, 1/3-cup plant milk, and 1 tbsp. unrefined coconut oil. Fold in ½ cup chopped strawberries.

Cook in an oiled pan, turning once. These will cook fairly quickly. Make a fruit compote, or add fruit butter to the top.

Noon Meal: Miso vegetable soup

Evening Meal: Soba noodles with green curry

Transitioning Vegan

BOOK 4

Introduction

Vegetarianism is nothing new. In fact, it has been around since, at least, 580 BC and was even a popular lifestyle choice for Pythagoras, who was an Ionian Greek philosopher and mathematician. Pythagoras was one of the first to admit that animals deserved to be treated well and people should try to abstain from consuming meat. These ideas of Pythagoras were not new, however, and in fact were the same traditions found in some earlier civilizations, like the ancient Egyptians.

Vegetarianism isn't just about animal cruelty, though that is a big reason for many people. It also provides a slew of health benefits that a meat filled diet just cannot give you. Vegetarian diets are actually really low in fat yet high in vegetables and fruits.

Maintaining a vegetarian diet also reduces the chance of suffering from food poison, which occurs millions of times a year due to spoiled meat. Studies have also shown that a meatless diet can help you shed those unwanted pounds. This has to do with several reasons, including replacing meat with more nutritious foods, such as whole grains, fresh fruits, fresh vegetables and beans.

Research has also shown that vegetarians are less likely to experience diseases, such as obesity, coronary heart disease, type two diabetes, high blood pressure and cancers related to diet.

In fact, living a vegan or vegetarian lifestyle can lower the amount of saturated fats while increasing the amount of healthy carbohydrates, fiber, potassium and magnesium you intake.

But what does this mean?

Well, reducing your intake of saturated fats will greatly improve your health, which is especially important if you deal with cardiovascular complications. Increasing healthy carbohydrates, which are naturally found in vegetables, will help prevent muscle mass burn, which essentially means you can maintain a healthy vegan/vegetarian lifestyle while still gaining muscle. And I'm sure you know that a diet high in fiber promotes healthier digestive tract. As for an increase in potassium and magnesium, well, these two vital minerals are essential for a healthy mind and body. Potassium helps to ensure the acidity and water in your body is properly balanced and it helps the kidneys get rid of harmful toxins. Studies have also shown that diets with an abundance of potassium can reduce the risk of cardiovascular dieses and cancer. Magnesium is an often overlook mineral/vitamin that is vital to the proper absorption of calcium. Dark greens, seeds and nuts are a few foods that are naturally high in magnesium.

Despite all the benefits that a vegan/vegetarian lifestyle has, trying to live in a meat eater's world can be more than a little difficult. Not only do you have to regularly explain to close minded people why you are a vegetarian (fielding questions and snide remarks left and right), but you also have to contend with the vegetarian diet, which can be more than a little daunting, especially for those new to this massive lifestyle change. After all, you are going against the traditional diet that is considered the traditional or normal way to live. Just turn on your television and after an hour you will have been bombarded with ads designed to entice the wild meat eating beast that lurks in all of use. But just because the initial transitioning is hard doesn't mean you cannot be successful.

That is where this vegetarian cookbook comes in handy. Not only does it provide the reader with 31 of the best recipes, it also gives you step-by-step instructions that even the most novice chef can follow.

A lot of people overlook the vegetarian lifestyle because they think it's too hard or takes too much time, which, let's face it, most people just don't have in their busy, fast-paced life. And while it is true that maintaining a vegetarian lifestyle can be a bit difficult at first, the benefits that you receive from living it is so worth it that you will wonder why you didn't come over to the plant-side sooner.

This vegetarian cookbook will help you in your journey into the wonderful world of vegetarianism. Inside this book, you will find recipes for every meal of the day, including breakfast, lunch and dinner. You will also find delicious smoothie, shake, juice and dessert recipes that won't break your vegetarian lifestyle.

So what are you waiting for? Start reading Chapter 1 now!

Chapter 1: Vegetarian Breakfast Recipes

The following breakfast recipes are designed to start your day off right while still maintaining your vegetarian lifestyle. Remember, breakfast is the most important meal of the day and you shouldn't skip it if at all possible.

Whole Wheat Pancakes

Serves: 4 to 5

Ingredients:

- 1 cup flour, whole wheat
- 1/3 cup wheat germ
- 2/3 cup flour, all-purpose
- 2 tablespoons brown sugar
- 1 teaspoon table salt
- ½ teaspoon baking soda
- 1 ½ teaspoon baking powder
- 2 large eggs, beaten
- 5 1/3 tablespoons butter, unsalted
- 2 ½ cups buttermilk

Directions:

Step 1: Combine the both flours, wheat germ, sugar, baking powder, baking soda and salt together in a mixing bowl.

Cut in the butter and continue to mix until it achieves a consistency similar to sand.

Step 2: Make a hole in the middle of the mixture. Pour the beaten eggs and buttermilk into the hole and mix until well combined.

Step 3: Use the batter to make the whole wheat pancakes as you normally would. Top with your favorite toppings, such as organic maple syrup or fruit.

Breakfast Casserole featuring Sweet Potatoes

Serves: 12

Ingredients:

- 1 8-ounce package vegetarian sausage, cooked
- ¼ cup butter, melted
- ½ cup water
- 4 cups sweet potatoes, shredded
- ½ cup onions, chopped finely
- 1 ½ 8-ounce package mozzarella/cheddar cheese blend
- 8 eggs, large
- 1 cup spinach, sliced
- 1 16-ounce container cottage cheese, small curd

Directions:

Step 1: Preheat the oven to 350-degrees and lightly grease a baking dish. Crumble the cooked vegetarian sausage into a bowl.

Step 2: Mix the melted butter and the shredded sweet potatoes together before spreading it into the baking dish from Step 1.

Step 3: Combine the cheese blend, eggs, sausage, onions and spinach together. Spread this mixture evenly over the butter/potato mixture.

Step 4: Place the baking dish in the oven and cook for about 20 minutes. Remove from the oven and let cool for a few minutes before serving.

Apple Wraps

Serves: 2

Ingredients:

- 2 whole wheat tortillas
- ¼ cup organic apple butter
- 2 cups green apples, cored/peeled/diced
- 1 cup rolled oats
- 1 teaspoon vanilla extract
- 1 tablespoon butter
- 1 ½ cup almond milk
- 1 teaspoon cinnamon
- 1/8 teaspoon salt
- ¼ cup organic raisins
- ¼ cup organic honey

Directions:

Step 1: Mix the honey, salt, cinnamon and raisins together. Add the apples and toss until coated.

Step 2: Melt the butter in a large saucepan. Add the coated apple and cook over medium heat for about 8 to 10 minutes. Make sure to stir occasionally. You want the apples to be tender.

Step 3: Stir in the milk and oatmeal before turning the heat down a bit and allowing to mixture to cook for about 5 minutes.

Step 4: Remove the saucepan from heat and stir in the vanilla. Evenly spread some organic apple butter on the tortillas before spooning the cooked mixture on top of the apple butter.

Step 5: Wrap the tortillas and serve warm.

Breakfast Green Smoothie

Serves: 1

Ingredients:

- 2 kale leaves
- 2 carrots
- 2 celery sticks
- 1 pear, remove core and slice into small pieces
- 1 knob ginger, small
- 2 cups baby spinach
- 1 tablespoons chia seeds
- 6 ice cubes

Directions:

Step 1: Place all ingredients into a blender and blend until smooth, which should be about 30 to 60 seconds.

Step 2: Pour the smoothie into a glass and enjoy.

Oatmeal and Blueberry Waffles

Serves: 3

Ingredients:

- 1 cup flour, whole wheat
- ½ teaspoon salt
- 1 tablespoon baking powder
- ¼ teaspoon allspice
- 1 cup oats, quick cooking
- 1/3 cup organic applesauce, unsweetened
- 1 ½ cups almond milk, unsweetened
- 2 tablespoons canola oil
- 3 tablespoons real maple syrup
- 1 teaspoon vanilla extract
- 1 ½ cup blueberries, frozen

Directions:

Step 1: Sift the baking powder, flour, allspice and salt together in a mixing bowl. Stir in the oats. Create a small well in the middle of the mixture and add the milk, applesauce, vanilla, oil and maple syrup into the whole. Mix until all ingredients are well combined.

Step 2: Allow the mixture to sit undisturbed for about 5 minutes. Gently fold the frozen blueberries into the mixture.

Step 3: Pour about ½ cup of the mixture into a heated waffle iron and cook until the waffle is done. Repeat with the remaining batter. Serve the waffles with your favorite toppings.

Chapter 2: Vegetarian Lunch Recipes

While the following vegetarian recipes are designed for lunchtime, you can make them at any time of the day.

Salsa and Black Bean Soup

Serves: 4

Ingredients:

- 2 cans black beans, drained and rinsed
- 1 cup salsa, chunky
- 1 ½ cup organic vegetable broth
- 1 teaspoon cumin
- 2 ½ tablespoons green onions, sliced

Directions:

Step 1: Pour the beans, vegetable broth, cumin and salsa into a blender and blend until the mixture is almost smooth.

Step 2: Pour the mixture into a large saucepan and place on the stove over medium heat. Heat until the mixture is completely heated.

Step 3: Divide the soup between 4 soup bowls and top with some sliced green onions.

Carrot and Lentil Soup

Serves: 2

Ingredients:

- 3 ounces red lentils
- 1 cube vegetable stock, crumbled
- 3 garlic cloves, sliced
- 2 carrots, cleaned and diced
- 2 teaspoons olive oil
- 1 onion, sliced finely
- 2 tablespoons parsley, chopped

Directions:

Step 1: Heat the oil in a saucepan. While the oil is heating, bring 1 liter of water to a boil.

Step 2: Add the chopped onions into the heated oil and fry for a few minutes. Add in the garlic and carrots.

Step 3: Carefully pour the boiling water into the saucepan with the onions, garlic and carrots. Stir in the vegetable stock cube and the lentils. Let cook for about 15 minutes.

Step 4: Remove the saucepan from heat and stir in the parsley. Spoon the soup into the bowls and serve while warm.

Tofu Lunch Scramble

Serves: 4

Ingredients:

- 1 14-ounce package tofu, rinsed
- 3 teaspoons canola oil, divided in half
- 1 teaspoon cumin
- 1 ½ teaspoons chili powder
- ½ teaspoon salt, divide in half
- ¾ cup corn
- 1 zucchini, diced
- 4 scallions, diced
- ½ cup salsa
- ½ cup shredded cheese
- ¼ cup cilantro, chopped

Directions:

Step 1: Place 1 ½ teaspoon of the oil into a large skillet. Warm the oil over medium heat. Stir in the tofu, cumin, chili powder and ¼ teaspoon of salt. Cook for about 6 minutes or until the tofu starts to turn a brownish color. When this occurs, transfer the mixture to a bowl.

Step 2: Mix in the remaining ingredients until everything is well combined. Divide the scramble between 4 dishes and serve immediately.

Fried Tofu and Mushrooms Served in Lettuce Cups

Serves: 6

Ingredients:

- 10 ¾ ounce shitake mushrooms, dried and chopped
- 1 tablespoon lime juice
- 2 tablespoons hoisin sauce
- 2 tablespoons roasted peanut oil
- 3 minced garlic cloves
- 1 Thai chili, seeds removed and diced
- 1 tablespoon minced ginger root
- 12 ounces tofu, drained and diced
- 12 lettuce leaves

Directions:

Step 1: Place a cup of hot water in a bowl and add the dried mushrooms. Let the mushrooms soak for about 10 minutes. Strain the liquid from the mushrooms and mix them the hoisin sauce.

Step 2: Coat a saucepan with the peanut oil and heat on the stove over medium heat. Place the mushrooms, ginger, chili and garlic into the heated pan and cook for a few minutes.

Step 3: Place the tofu into the pan and cook for several minutes. You want the tofu to have a light brown color.

Step 4: Spoon the cooked tofu mixture into the 12 lettuce leaves. Roll the leaves up and serve immediately.

Lunch Beans in a Crockpot

Serves: 4

Ingredients:

- 1 onion, diced
- 1 pound cannellini beans, dried
- 4 garlic cloves, minced
- 1 bay leaf
- 1 teaspoon thyme, dried
- ½ teaspoon salt, table or kosher
- 5 cups boiling water

Directions:

Step 1: Place the beans in a large pot filled with cold water. The beans should be completely covered by the water.

Let the beans soak for at least 6 hours but preferably overnight.

Step 2: Drain the beans from the water and place them inside crockpot. Stir in the diced onions, minced garlic cloves, bay leaf and thyme. Pour the boiling water overtop the ingredients. Place the cover on the crockpot and cook for 3 ½ hours.

Step 3: Add the salt and stir before placing the lid back n the crockpot and cooking and additional 15 minutes.

Tomato Basil Crockpot Soup

Serves: 4

Ingredients:

- 10 basil leaves, fresh
- 12 tomatoes, diced
- 6 ounce can tomato paste
- 1 tablespoon vegan butter
- ¼ teaspoon ground black pepper
- 1 tablespoon Italian seasoning
- 2 cups soy milk
- 2 tablespoons flour, whole wheat

Directions:

Step 1: Place the basil leaves, diced tomatoes, tomato paste and ground pepper into the crockpot.

Step 2: In a small bowl, whisk together the whole wheat flour and soy milk. Pour the mixture into the crockpot.

Step 3: Place the lid on the crockpot and cook on low for about 6 hours.

Step 4: Transfer the soup into a food processor and pulse for several seconds. You want the soup to have a little chunkiness to it. Place the soup make into the crockpot and keep warm until ready to serve.

Chapter 3: Vegetarian Dinner Recipes

If you find yourself searching for a vegetarian recipe to feed a large amount of people, simple double (or triple) the ingredients of these following dinner recipes, which will please both vegetarians and meat eaters a like.

Stuffed Peppers

Serves: 6

Ingredients:

- 2 cups brown rice, cooked
- 1 cup frozen corn, thawed
- 3 small tomatoes, diced
- 1 sweet onion, diced
- ¾ cup vegan cheese substitute
- 1/3 cup canned black beans, rinsed with water and drained
- 4 ¼ ounce ripe olives, chopped
- 1/3 cup canned red beans, rinsed with water and drained
- 3 garlic cloves, minced
- 4 fresh basil leaves, sliced thinly
- ½ teaspoon black pepper
- 1 teaspoon salt
- ¾ cup spaghetti sauce, meatless
- 6 sweet peppers, large
- ½ cup water

Directions:

Step 1: Mix the brown rice, tomatoes, corn, onion, cheese substitute, olives, beans, basil leaves, garlic cloves, salt and pepper together in a bowl.

Step 2: Cut the top of the sweet peppers off and remove the seeds inside. Stuff the peppers with the mixture from Step 1.

Step 3: Mix the meatless spaghetti sauce and water together. Pour half of this mixture into a crockpot. Place the stuffed peppers into the crockpot and pour the remaining water/sauce mixture on top.

Step 4: Place the lid on the crockpot and cook on low for 4 hours.

Cauliflower Tacos

Serves: 4 to 8

Ingredients:

- 1 cauliflower head
- 2 tablespoons olive oil, divided
- 1 can chickpeas
- 1 teaspoon salt, divided
- ¼ teaspoon cumin
- ¼ teaspoon chili powder
- 1 garlic clove, minced
- 2 cups cilantro, fresh
- 8 tortillas

Directions:

Step 1: Preheat the oven to 425-degrees. Cut the head of cauliflower into florets. Place the florets in a bowl and drizzle with 1 tablespoon olive oil and ½ teaspoon of salt. Spread the covered florets onto a baking sheet and bake for about 15 minutes. You want to brown the florets.

Step 2: While the florets are in the oven, mix the remaining salt, chickpeas, cumin and chili powder together in a bowl. Stir in the remaining olive oil. Spread the mixture onto a clean baking sheet and place in the oven for 15 minutes.

Step 3: Evenly divide the garlic and cilantro between the tortillas. Add ½ cup of the florets mixture and 1 teaspoon of the chickpea mixture to the tortillas. Roll the tortillas up and serve.

Bean Burgers Smokey-Style

Serves: 2

Ingredients:

- ½ cup sunflower seeds, coarsely chopped
- 1/3 cup oats, quick cooking
- ½ green bell pepper, diced
- 1 can pinto beans, drained and rinsed
- ½ cup hemp seeds
- 1 teaspoon chili powder
- 2 teaspoons salt
- 1 teaspoon paprika
- 1 tablespoon olive oil
- Salt and black pepper to taste
- Lettuce, tomatoes, onions and other toppings and/or condiments (optional)
- Hamburger buns, whole grain

Directions:

Step 1: Preheat the oven to 400-degrees. Mix the quick cooking oats with 2/3 cup of boiling water.

Step 2: Mix the hemp seeds, beans, bell pepper, olive oil and seasonings together in a bowl. Place the mixture in a food processor and process for several seconds.

Step 3: Transfer the pulsed mixture into a bowl and stir in the oatmeal and sunflower seeds.

Step 4: Coat the bottom of a baking sheet with olive oil. Scoop the mixture out of the bowl using a measuring cup.
Pat the mixture into a patty shape. Place the patty on the baking sheet.

Step 5: Place the baking sheet in the oven and bake for 15 minutes. Flip the patties and allow to bake for an additional 15 minutes.

Step 6: Serve the vegetarian burgers on whole grain bread with your desired toppings.

Rigatoni and Sautéed Vegetables

Serves: 2 to 4

Ingredients:

- 5 ½ cups rigatoni, cooked and drained according to the package instructions
- 1 eggplant, cut into bite-sized pieces
- 3 tablespoons olive oil
- 1 pint cherry tomatoes, cut in half
- 3 garlic cloves, thinly sliced
- ¼ cup fresh mint, torn into pieces
- Pinch of salt, table or kosher
- Pinch of black pepper

Directions:

Step 1: Place the oil in a skillet and heat over high heat. Add the pieces of eggplant, salt and pepper. Cook for about 10 minutes or until the eggplant develops a brown color. Make sure to stir the cooking eggplant occasionally.

Step 2: Stir in the halved tomatoes and garlic and cook for an additional 4 minutes. Add the cooked and drained rigatoni and the mint. Mix until all is well combined.

Step 3: Divide the meal between the serving bowls and enjoy.

Vegetarian Chili with a dash of Chocolate

Serves: 4

Ingredients:

- 1 ½ ounces chocolate, bittersweet
- 1 teaspoon salt
- 1 tablespoon olive oil
- 2 teaspoons cumin
- 1 garlic clove, minced
- 1 green pepper, diced
- 1 white onion, chopped finely
- 2 tomatoes, diced
- 2 cans kidney beans, drained and rinsed
- 2 cans chickpeas, drained and rinsed
- 5 cups vegetable broth

Directions:

Step 1: Place the oil in a large pot. Set the pot on the stove over high heat. Add the garlic, green pepper and onion.

Cook until the vegetables have begun to soften, which is generally about 5 minutes.

Step 2: Stir in the kidney beans, chickpeas, cumin, salt, tomatoes and vegetable broth. Let the mixture cook and bring it to a boil. Once it begins to boil, turn the heat to low, cover the pot and let the mixture simmer.

Step 3: Allow the mixture to cook for about an hour or until it starts to thicken. Stir in the chocolate and continue to cook until it has completely melted.

Step 4: Divide the vegetarian chili between the serving bowls and enjoy.

Vegetarian Sloppy Joes

Serves: 4

Ingredients:

- ½ cup quinoa
- 1 yellow onion, diced
- 1 tablespoon olive oil
- 1 ½ cup pinto beans, drained and rinsed
- ½ green pepper, diced
- 1 can tomato sauce
- 1 tablespoon soy sauce
- 1 tomato, diced
- 2 teaspoons chili powder
- ¼ teaspoon oregano, dried
- ½ teaspoon paprika
- Rolls, whole grain

Directions:

Step 1: In a small pot, mix 1 cup of water with the quinoa. Bring the mixture to a boil before reducing the heat and covering the pot. Let the mixture simmer for about 15 minutes.

Step 2: Place the olive oil in a skillet. Sauté the diced onion for a few minutes. Stir in the green pepper and continue to sauté until the vegetables are tender.

Step 3: Stir in the remaining ingredients except for the whole grain rolls. Let the ingredients cook for about 5 minutes. Remove the mixture from heat and let sit for an additional 5 minutes.

Step 4: Stir in the mixture from step 1 and let sit for another 5 minutes. Scoop the mixture onto the whole grain rolls and serve with a side of your favorite vegetables or salad.

Pad Thai Noodles

Serves: 3 to 4

Ingredients:

- 1 package rice noodles, cooked according to the directions on the package
- ½ cup peanut butter
- 1 cup coconut milk
- 2 garlic cloves, minced
- 1 tablespoon ginger, fresh
- ¼ cup lime juice
- ½ teaspoon salt, table or kosher
- 1 teaspoon chili sauce
- ½ teaspoon peanut oil
- 1 cup tofu
- 1 red pepper, diced
- 2 cups shitake mushrooms, sliced
- 1 cup snow peas
- 1 cup broccoli florets
- 1 cup baby bok choy, chopped
- ½ cup peanuts, roasted
- Olive oil

Directions:

Step 1: Mix the peanut butter, coconut milk, ginger, salt, garlic, peanut oil, lime juice and chili sauce together. Set to the side for the moment.

Step 2: In a pan, heat the olive oil. Add the tofu and cook until it is brown on all sides. Remove the tofu from the pan and set to the side for the moment.

Step 3: Add 1 teaspoon of olive oil to the pan and sauté the mushrooms, broccoli florets, snow peas and bell pepper for about 10 minutes.

Step 4: Stir in the bok choy and browned tofu. Cook for an additional 2 minutes.

Step 5: Divide the cooked noodles between the serving dishes. Add the browned tofu and bok choy. Drizzle the mixture from Step 1 over the top and garnish with roasted peanuts.

Vegetarian Pizza

Serves: Makes 2 9x18-inches pizzas

Ingredients:

- 2 teaspoons red peppers, diced
- 2 eggplants, diced
- ½ cup olive oil, extra virgin
- 2 pounds frozen pizza dough
- 3 cups shredded mozzarella vegan substitute
- 1 ½ cups tomato sauce
- Fresh basil
- Pinch salt, table or kosher
- Pinch black pepper
- Sweet potatoes

Directions:

Step 1: Turn the grill on and let heat at a medium to high temperature.

Step 2: Toss all the vegetables with ¼ cup of the olive oil. Season with salt and pepper.

Step 3: Grill the coated vegetables in batches until they are soft but still have a bit of crunch to them. Place the grilled vegetables to the side.

Step 4: Roll the pizza dough out to make 2 9x18-inch pizzas that are about 1/8-inch thick.

Step 5: Brush one side of the pizza with 1 tablespoon of olive oil. Do the same for the second pizza. Season the pizza with salt and pepper. Place the pizzas, oil-side down, onto the grill. Grill for about 9 minutes.

Step 6: Repeat Step 5 with the opposite side of the pizzas.

Step 7: Evenly spread the pizza sauce over one side of each pizza. Top with the vegan cheese substitute and grilled vegetables. Close the lid of the grill and let the cheese substitute melt. Garnish with fresh basil before cutting the pizzas into slices.

Chapter 4: Vegetarian Smoothie, Shakes and Juice Recipes

The following smoothie, shakes and juice recipes can be used as a meal substitute or for when you're craving something but don't want a big meal. In fact, the following recipes work great as an on-the-go breakfast meal when you just don't have the time to prepare and sit down to eat a traditional breakfast meal.

Banana and Ginger Smoothie

Serves: 1

Ingredients:

- 1 ripe banana, sliced
- 1 tablespoon honey
- 1 cup vanilla vegan yogurt
- ½ teaspoon grated ginger

Directions:

Step 1: Place all 4 ingredients into a blender and blend until the mixture is smooth. Pour the smoothie into a tall glass and enjoy.

Purple Power Smoothie

Serves: 1

Ingredients:

- ½ cup blueberries
- 1 ¼ cup milk, soy
- ½ banana
- 1 teaspoon vanilla extract
- 2 teaspoons sugar

Directions:

Step 1: Place all the ingredients into a blender and blend until smooth. Pour the smoothie into a glass and enjoy.

Chocolate and Cherry Shake

Serves: 1

Ingredients:

- 12 ounces soy milk
- 2 scoops protein powder, chocolate flavor
- 2 cups cherries, pitted
- 1 tablespoon walnuts
- 1 cup baby spinach
- 1 tablespoon dark cocoa powder
- 1 tablespoon ground flax

Directions:

Step 1: Add all ingredients into a blender and blend until smooth. Transfer the shake into a glass and enjoy.

Green Detox Smoothie

Serves: 1

Ingredients:

- 1 kiwi, peeled
- ½ cup pineapple, chopped
- 1 cup coconut water
- Handful baby spinach
- ½ avocado, peeled and chopped
- 1 teaspoon coconut oil

Directions:

Step 1: Add all ingredients into a blender and blend until smooth. Transfer the detox smoothie into a glass and enjoy.

Berry Strawberry Smoothie

Serves: 1

Ingredients:

- 2 cups strawberries, stems removed
- 2 basil springs
- 1 handful mint
- 1 ripe banana
- ½ cup apple juice
- 1 teaspoon honey

Directions:

Step 1: Add all ingredients into a blender and blend until smooth. Transfer the shake into a glass and enjoy.

Pumpkin Pie Smoothie

Serves: 1

Ingredients:

- 1 cup almond milk
- 1 cup pumpkin puree
- 1 teaspoon agave nectar
- 1 red apple, cored
- 2 teaspoons cinnamon
- Handful cranberries, dried

Directions:

Step 1: Add all ingredients into a blender and blend until smooth. Transfer the shake into a glass and enjoy.

Antioxidant Boost Smoothie

Serves: 1

Ingredients:

- ½ cup acia berry puree
- ½ cup pomegranate arils
- 1 ripe banana
- ½ cup blueberries
- 8 ounces almond milk

Directions:

Step 1: Add all ingredients into a blender and blend until smooth. Transfer the shake into a glass and enjoy.

Golden Delicious Juice

Serves: 1

Ingredients:

- 4 stalks celery
- 2 carrots
- ½ cucumber
- 1 pear
- ½ cup beetroot
- Sprinkle ginger, diced

Directions:

Step 1: Place all ingredients into a blender. Blend for several seconds or until the ingredients are smooth.

Step 2: Pour the juice into a glass and enjoy immediately.

Chapter 5: Vegetarian Dessert Recipes

Yes, even vegetarians can make and enjoy delicious desserts while still maintaining their vegetarian lifestyle. And these yummy dessert recipes prove just that!

Chocolate and Banana Mousse

Serves: 4

Ingredients:

- 1 cup semi-sweet chocolate chips
- 2 bananas, ripe
- 10 ounce tofu, silken soft
- 3 tablespoons brown sugar
- 1 teaspoon vanilla extract
- 1 teaspoon raspberry vinegar
- ¼ teaspoon salt

Directions:

Step 1: In a microwave safe bowl, melt the chocolate chips.

Step 2: Place half the banana and the tofu into a blender and blend until the two ingredients are smooth. Add the other half of the banana and blend until smooth.

Step 3: Add in the brown sugar, raspberry vinegar, salt and vanilla extract and blend until smooth. Transfer the melted chocolate chips into the blender and blender once more.

Step 4: Scoop the mixture out of the blender and into an air tight container. Place the container in the fridge and chill for at least 3 hours before consuming.

Simple Fruit Cocktail Cake

Serves: 6

Ingredients:

- 9 ounce package yellow cake mix
- 1 can fruit cocktail packed in light syrup

Directions:

Step 1: Preheat the oven to 350-degrees. Light grease the inside of a baking pan that measures 9x9-inches.

Step 2: Drain the fruit cocktail, pouring the syrup into a mixing bowl. Add the cake mix and combined until well mixed.

Step 3: Gently mix in the fruit cocktail. Spread the mixture into the prepared baking pan. Place the pan in the oven and bake for about 45 minutes.

Biscotti al Pistachio

Serves: 2 dozen cookies

Ingredients:

- 500 grams raw pistachios
- 1 teaspoon vanilla extract
- 200 grams white sugar
- 1 ½ teaspoon lemon zest
- 1 tablespoon honey
- Powdered sugar

Directions:

Step 1: Place the pistachios into a food processor and pulse until they are finely chopped.

Step 2: Transfer the chopped pistachios into a mixing bowl. Stir in the white sugar, lemon zest, vanilla extract and honey. This is the dough.

Step 3: Roll the dough into small balls and cover them with powdered sugar. Place the dough onto a parchment paper-lined cookie sheet.

Step 4: Place the cookie sheets into a oven preheated at 350-degrees. Bake for 16 to 18 minutes.

Pumpkin and Pear Dessert Bread

Serves: 1 loaf

Ingredients:

- 1 cup all-purpose flour
- 1 ¼ cup white sugar
- 1 cup whole wheat flour
- 2 teaspoon cinnamon
- 2 teaspoon baking powder
- 1 teaspoon baking soda
- ¼ teaspoon table or kosher salt
- ½ cup milk, almond, coconut or soy
- ¾ cup pumpkin puree
- ½ cup vegetable oil
- 1 15-ounce can pears, drained and diced
- 1 teaspoon real vanilla extract

Directions:

Step 1: Preheat the oven to 350-degrees. Spray a 9-inch loaf pan with cooking spray. Set the pan to the side for the moment.

Step 2: Mix the sugar, baking powder, baking soda, cinnamon, salt and flour together. Place to the side for the moment.

Step 3: In a second mixing bowl, combined the vanilla, milk, oil and pumpkin puree. Add in the flour mixture from step 2. Fold in the pears.

Step 4: Pour the batter into the prepared pan from Step 1. Place the loaf pan in the preheated oven and bake for 55 minutes or until a toothpick inserted into the center of the bread comes out clean.

Step 5: Let the bread cool for several minutes before cutting and serving.

CPSIA information can be obtained
at www.ICGtesting.com
Printed in the USA
LVHW080517220321
682038LV00014B/377